The Ultimate Twin Dad Survival Guide

Preparation Tips, Hacks, and Sanity Savers

Scott Southworth

Copyright © 2025

All Rights Reserved

ISBN:

Dedication

To my wife, who has walked every step of this journey with me, thank you for always pushing me to reach for the stars. Thank you for being the most amazing person in my life who always roots for me and my crazy dreams, like writing a book to help other Dads navigate the beginning of their twin journey.

To my daughters, thank you for filling my heart with an abundance of joy each and every day. Giving me the strength and passion to always move forward. I hope that I am able to show you all the love that you deserve from a Father.

To all the Dads out there that are reading this book, thank you for taking a step towards being the best Dad you can be. Our society will greatly benefit from more amazing fathers. I hope this book helps you understand and prepare for the Dad twin life.

Disclaimer

The suggestions and recommendations that I offer in this book are based solely on my personal experience with my twins and countless hours of research. Please note, that in this book, there could be inaccuracies or tips which are provided which have no medical standing. I want to be upfront with you as the reader that I am just a dad wanting to help others navigate this brand-new world that is the twin dad chaos. I have made effort to ensure that the information in this book is correct at printing, while this publication is designed to provide accurate information, I assume no responsibility for any errors, omissions, other inconsistencies in this book as well as any actions you take. I hereby disclaim any liability to any party for damage, disruption, or loss that may result in any error or accident from your actions.

The information in this provided in this book is for informational purposes only and is not intended for any medical, legal, or financial advice. As a disclosure, I am not a doctor or in any part of the medical industry, so be sure to consult with your wife or spouse's OBGYN doctor, as well as your children's pediatrician for any and all medical related matters. I also am not a lawyer or financial consultant, so should you want to discuss any topics or issues that arise in those areas of specialty, please seek professional help. My opinions with regards to all of these issues are just that, my opinion.

I fully understand that each family is different, each pregnancy is different, everyone's health is different, and everyone's situation is different. You may have a better experience than I did or a worse experience. This book outlines what I personally went through and provides what worked best in our situation. I do hope that some of the information which is broken down in this book can help you be the best TWIN DAD and husband /spouse you can be. Take everything in life with a grain of salt.

Table of Contents

Chapter One: Finding Out About Twins 1

Chapter Two: Pregnancy and Pregnancy Nutrition 7

Chapter Three: Getting the House and Family Ready 14

Chapter Four: Setting up for You and Your Wife 29

Chapter Five: Closer to Birth 31

Chapter Six: Hospital and Delivery 35

Chapter Seven: Babies' First Moments 43

Chapter Eight: NICU Time 47

Chapter Nine: Coming Home from the Hospital 53

Chapter Ten: Formulas 56

Chapter Eleven: Pediatrician and What to Expect 59

Chapter Twelve: When Does It Get Easier? 62

Our Story 66

Random Advice and Food for Thought 71

About the Author

Scott Southworth is a proud father of twin girls and a first-time author whose journey into fatherhood inspired him to write The Ultimate Twin Dad Survival Guide. As a debut author, Scott brings a fresh, honest, and heartfelt perspective to parenting multiples infusing his writing with practical advice, humor, and real-life experience.

Motivated by the chaos and joy of raising twins, Scott created this guide to support and encourage fellow dads navigating the unique challenges of twin parenthood. His hands-on insights, thoughtful preparation tips, and relatable storytelling make this book an indispensable resource for new and expecting fathers of multiples.

When he's not busy juggling diapers and bottles, Scott enjoys spending time with his family, building meaningful memories, and helping other parents step confidently into their roles.

Chapter One: Finding Out About Twins

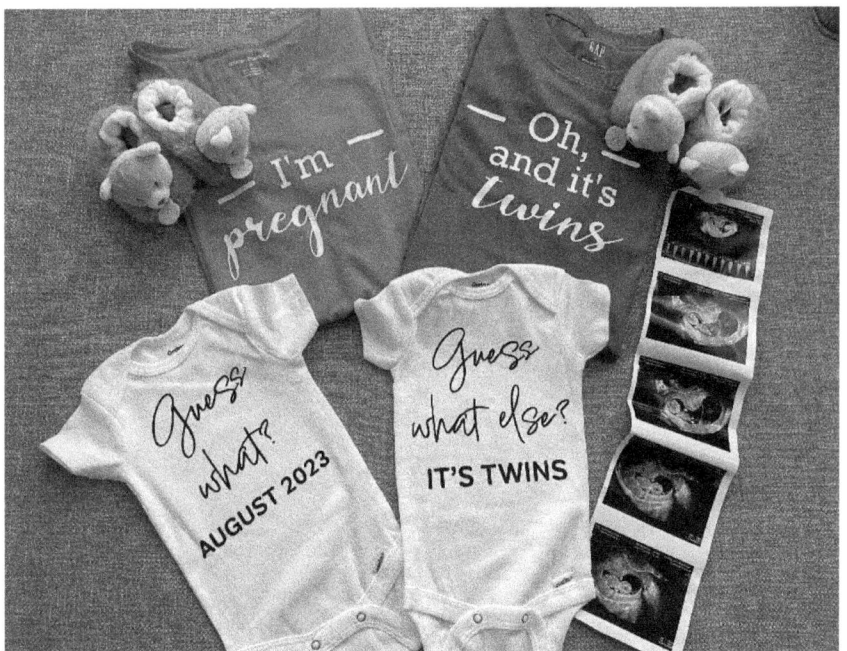

YOU ARE HAVING TWINS! Welcome to the Twin Dad Group.

Nothing can truly prepare you for the reality of twins, but this book is designed to help you navigate this surprise through the eyes of a fellow twin dad. As I go into further detail within the "Our Story" section, you will see that my wife and I knew that twins were a possibility. However it was much more difficult at the beginning than either of us anticipated. If you already have any children, don't be fooled, having twins is a whole different ball game. The lack of sleep, the crying, the responsibility, etc. As the man in the relationship, it is our responsibility to be the leader. That's our job. What does it mean to be the leader of your house?

The head of the household is one which is the rock and the foundation of the family. This means stepping up, making money, taking care of the house, being the spiritual leader of the family, buying what is needed, helping out with the kids, and doing what needs to be done to help your wife/significant other as much as possible. But more on this later…

When you find out you're having twins, there are two reactions:

The first reaction is "TWINS, WHAT?!" followed by a lot of excitement. You start thinking about what genders they are and how busy you'll be. You'll start daydreaming of playing with them and teaching them everything you know.

Then the second reaction is one of a little bit more nervousness, you think to yourself, "Oh my gosh, multiple kids at one time!" A little bit of panic starts to creep in. Don't worry, this book has a lot of information for you on how to survive and ultimately thrive as a twin dad. Life may just be a little more chaotic than you are used to; however, as my wife likes to describe it, it is joyful chaos.

How did this happen, and what kind of twins are they?

Having twins that develop naturally is just that – Natural. Either you have one fertilized egg split, and then you have identical twins, meaning the same genetic information for both babies. Your twins will look the same, but they will still have two different personalities. You can also have Fraternal twins. This means that MOM's ovaries drop two eggs (or more), and those eggs are fertilized. Your twins will not look alike or have the same genetics.

There can also be medical ways in order to conceive twins or multiples. If you are having trouble conceiving and getting medical help, chances are you have already been told that multiple kids are a possibility. Medically, you typically have a few options for help conceiving.

Hormone Therapy: This can be done using a hormone called Clomiphene. This will help MOM release multiple eggs while they ovulate. This is typically the cheapest of the medical assistance options; however, our doctor made it abundantly clear that twins (or more) were a high possibility. This is the direction that my wife and I proceeded with first. My wife was able to get pregnant during the first ovulation cycle with this method, so we did not have to proceed with the following methods.

Next, you have "IUI" or Intrauterine insemination, or as I call it, the "turkey baster." Basically, DAD would provide a "sample" to the doctors in the office. Then, at the right time of the month during MOM's ovulation, an appointment would be made, and the doctor would place DAD's sample where it needs to go in order to help provide a better chance of conception. This is typically how you can have one child at a time, unless the eggs split and there are identical twins. This procedure is in the middle ground of cost. My wife and I had this choice along with the Clomiphene; however, we went with the Clomiphene mainly for the cost. At that time, we were having a hard time emotionally, not getting pregnant, so we decided it was worth just trying the cheapest option first for one month and then moving on from there.

Lastly, you have "IVF" or In Vitro Fertilization. IVF is pretty rough on the females. It starts with retrieving an egg from MOM and a sample from DAD. Fertilizing the egg in the medical office. MOM would be required to go on hormones, and the doctors implant the fertilized egg in her uterus. This is very expensive to do, but it can work a lot of the time. Unfortunately, some people are unsuccessful conceiving this way and have to go through this procedure multiple times. If you're considering this, your doctor will go over the success rates with you.

The way my wife and I conceived the twins caused us to have what's referred to as DI/DI twins. There are a few different types of twins and each one has a risk factor associated with them, but DI/DI is the least concerning.

DI/DI – Dichorionic Diamniotic – This means that each twin has its own placenta and amniotic sac. I will note that all fraternal twins are Di/Di, but some identicals can be as well. This is the most ideal type of twins with the least pregnancy risk involved.

Mono/Di - Monochorionic Diamniotic – This means identical twins that share a placenta, but have a separate amniotic sac.

Mono/Mono - Monochorionic Monoamniotic twins – This means they are identical twins that share a placenta and an amniotic sac.

Conjoined: This means two babies born physically connected together. This is very rare and when the embryo forms identical twins, but only partially splits apart.

The Ultimate Twin Dad Survival Guide

When will MOM start to feel the twins?

Typically, MOM will start to feel the twins around 15 to 16 weeks in little flutters, and feel them more around the 20-24 week mark. These movements are so fun. It helps MOM connect emotionally with the babies a little bit more as the pregnancy becomes a little bit more real to you.

Are there possible complications?

There are many possible complications with a twin pregnancy. One big one is called twin-to-twin transfusion syndrome (**TTTS**). TTTS only occurs with identical twins that share the same placenta in the womb. It is an abnormal circumstance of how the blood vessels are attached to the babies. It is considered rare, but it happens more than doctors discuss. The basic idea is that one baby (the donor) will transfer blood to the other twin (the recipient). The donor twin will have stunted growth because it is giving the recipient twin blood and nutrients. In turn, the recipient twin will have too much blood flow and nutrients, which can cause heart trouble and other health-related complications.

Preeclampsia is another pregnancy risk. Preeclampsia is characterized by high blood pressure (hypertension) and protein in the urine (proteinuria) that develops during the 2nd half of the pregnancy. This high blood pressure for MOM can, in turn, cause low blood flow for the babies, which is a dangerous situation.

Stunted growth because of an umbilical cord blood flow issue can also be a major problem. The doctors referred to this as IGUR

(Intrauterine Growth Restriction). This is the condition where a fetus grows slower than expected during the pregnancy. This is what happened for our fraternal twins. For some reason, one twin sometimes does not get good blood flow through the umbilical cord. This will result in slow growth because they will not receive the correct nutrients that they need. Think of this like a hose, when you open the nozzle, it will flow in a steady stream. When there is intermediate or absent flow, it is as if the hose is kinked or you have your finger over the nozzle, so the amount of water / and in this case, nutrients, are obstructed. The last type of umbilical flow issues would be that it has reversed, which means that the baby is losing the nutrients, and is an automatic trigger for delivery (no matter how far along MOM is). Our twins were born right before 32 weeks because the doctors determined it was more beneficial for the babies to come out and get the nutrients, they needed within the NICU rather than stay in and cause stress on the babies and their growth.

Chapter Two: Pregnancy and Pregnancy Nutrition

Pregnancy is a crazy whirlwind of emotions for everyone involved. This topic alone could be a whole book. Let's just go through some of the biggest topics.

Pregnancy Emotions

The ups and downs of pregnancy are so confusing. She will be happy and feeling good, and then you sneeze and she is mad at you for sneezing too loudly. Maybe she is mad at you because of a dream she had, or happy tears because she saw a cute dog on TV. Nothing is off limits! Just keep that in mind and stay calm. If she's getting crazy and you match that energy, it won't be fun for either of you. My wife and I have a fun relationship so I was able to call out the pregnancy emotions and laugh at her when it happened. Sometimes she won't be willing to blame the emotions on the pregnancy, but you will know. Learn to pick your battles and words wisely, and **ultimately** be patient. A lot of these emotions are because her hormones are going crazy, creating new life, and she does not have a choice in how her body produces the hormones.

Scott Southworth

Morning Sickness

This can be a big one, but here are some things to consider about it.

It isn't just in the morning. Morning sickness can happen all day or at any point in the day. When it happens in the morning, it is because you don't have food when you're sleeping, so when MOM wakes up she needs to eat something that will help calm her stomach. Many of the times, it typically happens in the morning where the MOM will feel nauseous or clammy and this would result in throwing up or just having a really hard time with acid reflux.

What causes it? Ultimately, it is hormonal changes and lower blood sugar. Though you can't do anything about hormonal changes, there is some good news that you CAN do something about the blood sugar. Helping mom out with morning sickness will greatly benefit both of you.

So what was our helpful secret? FRUIT! Low blood sugar is just that, lower sugar in your blood. Have you ever not eaten for a while and gotten a little shaky, hangry, and felt sick? Well, that is what is happening in this case. So, a suggestion is to find a fruit that MOM likes. My wife liked grapes, easy on the stomach with a good amount of natural sugar in them. As soon as she woke up, it was straight to the kitchen for a big handful. This helped tremendously. This trick isn't 100% fool proof, but it works well. Also, don't forget to keep track of eating times throughout the day. Like I said earlier, it isn't only in the morning. My wife would carry snacks in her purse and work bag, which helped when she was out and about and started to feel nauseous. Protein bars and bags of mixed nuts helped tremendously.

Pregnancy Nutrition

First and foremost, always listen to your doctor's advice. There will be a lot of doctor visits, and they will know your situation best. You can do a lot in the way of nutrition that will not only help your babies grow, but also help MOM feel less physically bad as her pregnancy progresses. We already know that people who eat "healthy" look and feel better, but what some people don't realize is that the nutrients in your food also go to your babies as well. So here are a few tips:

A good prenatal vitamin. Ask your doctor which one they suggest. A good prenatal will have all of the recommended dosages of vitamins and minerals. Here you're looking for the basics like iron, calcium, vitamin D, but also folic acid in the form of Methylated Folate. About 40% of our population cannot convert regular "Folic Acid" to its usable form in our bodies, so getting it in this form will allow the MOM's body to process it. At this point, most of the good prenatal vitamins already have this, but make sure to read the label on the back of the bottle before you purchase.

The doctors will tell you to stay away from certain foods. MOM will have to give up sandwich meats, sushi and raw fish, and even steak that is undercooked. Only well-done steaks are recommended during pregnancy. The doctors even suggest staying away from regular mayo as this has uncooked eggs. Luckily for this one, I was able to find some vegan mayo that was a fair substitute for my wife. It was even made with avocado oil as a healthier oil instead of canola or soybean oils. Instead of turkey meat for sandwiches, I cooked fresh chicken for her and made chicken melt sandwiches. You can easily substitute some of your favorite foods for those that are healthier, you just need to get a little creative at times.

MOM will get some weird food cravings. My wife wanted hot and spicy things. Habanero hot sauce type of things. Things she used to eat she no longer wanted, and foods she never ate sounded SO good to her. Pregnancy messes with smells and tastes A LOT. Your wife may want pickle ice cream, or a chicken sandwich with a large bowl of pickles – bigger than the sandwich, or potato chips with fruit on top. Each mom is different. Do your best to help out, but you also get to keep her in check a little bit. Eating healthy is very important during pregnancy. Keep track of any funny food combinations that she comes up with. These will be funny stories to tell later.

Smells – This is a funny one. Sometimes new smells are good and some are bad, or MOM can't stand to be around normal odors you have in your house. For instance, one time I sprayed some bathroom spray in the house and it made my wife throw up for 20 minutes. I felt really bad for that one since it was directly caused by my actions. I had to apologize, but she forgave me. It is a funny story now, looking back, but it was not very funny at the time. I would always feel bad if my wife had a bad reaction to other smells, but I just try to remember that "it's all part of the ride" of pregnancy. The funny thing is that she now eats some of the foods that she ate during pregnancy. This makes me wonder if somehow it permanently changes how MOMs think about the food they eat.

The Ultimate Twin Dad Survival Guide

MOM will need a slight increase in calories depending on her starting weight. Remember, what nutrition MOM eats, babies also eat. At the beginning, MOM won't need as much because the babies are small, but nearing the 3rd trimester and those last few weeks to the finish line is where the babies will put on some weight. During this whole time, I kept reminding my wife that the babies are still small at the end - ours were only 2 and 3 pounds each. It is very natural for the MOM to gain extra weight, although some women stay fairly thin through the whole pregnancy.

MOM will lose a little bit of weight during delivery and recovery, but everything else is normal weight which she will have to try to lose later. Keep in mind that this is about the babies, so don't focus too much on your wife adding weight, she has to, but there is no reason to gain 50-100 extra pounds during the pregnancy.

Doing exercise and walking is a good thing. It's a good benefit to keep MOM's body moving while she can for her health. If you have visited a fertility doctor, there might be stricter restrictions on physical exercise during the first trimester compared to if you conceive naturally. As the babies grow, physical exercise will become harder. Growing multiple babies is very exhausting, some say it's like running a marathon. Make sure you listen to your doctor's advice on exercise and physical activity. The MOM is most likely going to have multiple doctors visits to her normal OBGYN and high-risk clinics. The doctors may put MOM on bed rest at some point if there are any complications that arise with the pregnancy.

Like I just mentioned, there will be lots of doctor visits. More than with a singleton. This is because with multiples come more risks, not only for MOM's health, but also for the babies. MOM will end up visiting a high-risk doctor in addition to her OBGYN at some point. These doctors do ultrasounds for measurements of the baby's growth. They will be able to see if the babies are having any growth restriction problems or blood flow problems. They will also be able to hear the heartbeat. These visits are crucial because it is good to detect early if something is a problem.

At this point, it's definitely worth mentioning that the high-risk doctors can be "jumpy" when it comes to seeing problems with the babies (usually growth or blood flow). However, they really do care about the health of the babies and want you to have a good pregnancy. So, if they feel that something may be wrong, they will let you know what to do next.

If the doctors see a problem with the pregnancy, they will go over different options of how to proceed, and may potentially suggest having an abortion of one of the babies to ensure that the other baby has a more viable option for the remainder of the pregnancy. As wild as that sounds, they call it "selective reduction" to try to make it sound better. Whatever your stance is on this, you are killing a human life if you do it. The high-risk doctors told my wife that she had this option, and they suggested it since our babies had growth restriction issues. Following that visit, we requested not to be affiliated with that doctor anymore. It was sad to hear him easily suggest it like it was nothing. Needless to say, both of our babies were born and are thriving to this day. We couldn't imagine our life without one of them, they both are so amazing.

The Ultimate Twin Dad Survival Guide

The final issue I'll talk about in this pregnancy section is vaccines for MOM while pregnant. Whether MOM takes any (Flu, DTAP, etc.) it is <u>ALWAYS</u> up to you. The doctors are supposed to try to get you to take shots, even making you feel guilty or bad if you say no or want to wait. The goal is to do what is best for the health and safety of the babies. There are lots of stories out there of moms getting shots and having miscarriages. But there are also lots of stories of times when nothing happens. You will have to weigh the pros and cons of each and make the choice. For my wife and I, we chose no vaccines because we didn't want any more question marks with our already at-risk pregnancy. I talk about it a little more in the "Our Story" section, but I'll mention that since we had a fairly risky pregnancy from the beginning, we did not want to jeopardize anyone's health by introducing any foreign substances into the mix.

Chapter Three: Getting the House and Family Ready

As the pregnancy is progressing, now is the time to start sharing the good news to family and friends. Though this is an exciting time, it can also be new territory for families with toddlers in the house. Be sure to prep your other children, as this will be critical for them to start to understand what is about to happen. It helps your older children emotionally and allows them to grasp that there are new babies coming and to be excited that they will now be a big sister or brother. Breaking the news to older children can be complicated. Do your best to make it a fun experience for them. It's your job to help them try to navigate their feelings, not only here, but as they grow up. Most kids are naturally excited, but you can help them get excited if they aren't.

After telling your other children, you can break the news to other relatives and friends. Sharing that you are pregnant with twins will light up every single room you enter. There is so much excitement for the double blessings. Double the onesies, and double the diapers. As you share the news with everyone, remind them that you will definitely need some help when the babies are born, to get them mentally ready to provide some help to you. Get as much help as you can. Many people will offer help even though at first you may not know what you need, I'll tell you right now, you will need to sleep, so having someone help with dishes and cleaning bottles or cleaning is going to be so helpful. Though you may not want a ton of people at your home when the babies arrive, collecting diapers/wipes prior to delivery or setting up a meal train can be super beneficial. For example, your mom might be willing to bring food for you on Mondays and Fridays and your best friend loves to make crock pot recipes and can freeze you a meal for Wednesdays or Saturdays. Literally, this was a lifesaver those first few weeks after the twins came home.

It is also important to start planning ahead to take time off of work. It is critical that you try to take as much time off of work that you can in order to help take care of the babies when they come home. MOM will struggle a lot by herself, and she NEEDS your help. It will be all hands on deck when the babies come home (more than you anticipate).

If you're not able to take time off work, then you will need to arrange and ask family or friends for additional help. You may also need to hire a nanny. I hired someone to come to the house two days a week who would help us with feeding, changing diapers, cleaning bottles, etc. As much as the extra hands were helpful for cleaning, we really brought her on because we needed the sleep. One of us would stay with the nanny to help out with one of the twins and the other would get some uninterrupted sleep. Nannies can be expensive, not everyone is financially able to hire someone to come in to help, but it seriously helped us out.

I was blessed with my job and was able to take a little under 4 months off work. I'm not telling you to do that, but more to remind you to take the time off that you are given in order to help out. Half of my time off was paid vacation, and the other half was not. We live in a high cost of living area, so those unpaid times were sad seeing all that money go out of our accounts without the extra income. Plus, it was the holidays and we had to buy Christmas presents for our extended family, AND our refrigerator and microwave both decided it was time to stop working and required us to buy new ones. Thankfully, we had funds in our emergency fund account to help offset these costs, which leaves me in the next section of finances.

Finances

Getting your finances in order is a must!! You are the leader of the household. You got this!! Kids are expensive, let alone having two at the same time. Start saving money as soon as you find out you are having babies. Don't eat out as much, try to pick up extra shifts at work if you can, and save that money! You will need as much as you can accumulate because you will need to buy wipes, diapers, clothing, formula, food for you and your wife, rent, other bills, etc. It is a big list, but don't worry, I have you covered with an easy-to-calculate sheet below for how much you will want to have set aside.

Pull out a piece of paper. Start writing down the things that you know about first, per month. Then write down baby products, and add in some miscellaneous expenses, because things always happen that are not expected. Some of the things for the babies will probably be gifted to you at a baby shower. However, it is still a good idea to calculate the finances with baby products just in case. Below is a small example of what it should look like:

Rent = $1500

Phone = $200

Internet = $80

Electric = $100

Gas = $25

Adult Food = $500

Diapers = $150

Formula + Baby Water = $250

Baby Clothes = $100

Gas for Car = $100

Miscellaneous = $500

Nanny = $18-22/ hour

House Cleaning Maid (if you want) = $250

Example Total: $3,655 plus for 1 month

The above example is just a snapshot idea of, honestly, what you should be doing on a monthly basis anyway. Doing this will give you a good idea of your expenses for 1 month, and then you can multiply that by 2 or more if you need. Granted, this is if you are unpaid while off of work, but you should still have an emergency fund of cash just in case something unexpected happens. Most financial "gurus" will say you should have 3-6 months' worth of emergency fund, like this, set aside at all times.

Setting Up the House

Furniture

The next item to discuss about getting the house ready is furniture. There is no need to go crazy expensive with this, just find things that work for you and that you like. Keep in mind, you don't have to have the entire nursery set up as soon as the babies arrive. Most of the time, they will be in a bassinet close to you for the first 6 months. Below are some of the key pieces of furniture that were a MUST for us.

Bassinets

You have two options here for twins – singles or doubles. From experience and my personal opinion, I would recommend going with two single bassinets. We originally bought a double bassinet prior to the twin's arrival; however, once the girls came home and they started sleeping side by side, one would wiggle while sleeping, which would wake the other one up. We ended up buying a single bassinet and put one baby in that and put the other baby on one side of the double bassinet so that they wouldn't shake each other awake. I will mention, however, that we did like having the double bassinet available during the day and placed our twins in there during their wake windows so that they could still be next to each other.

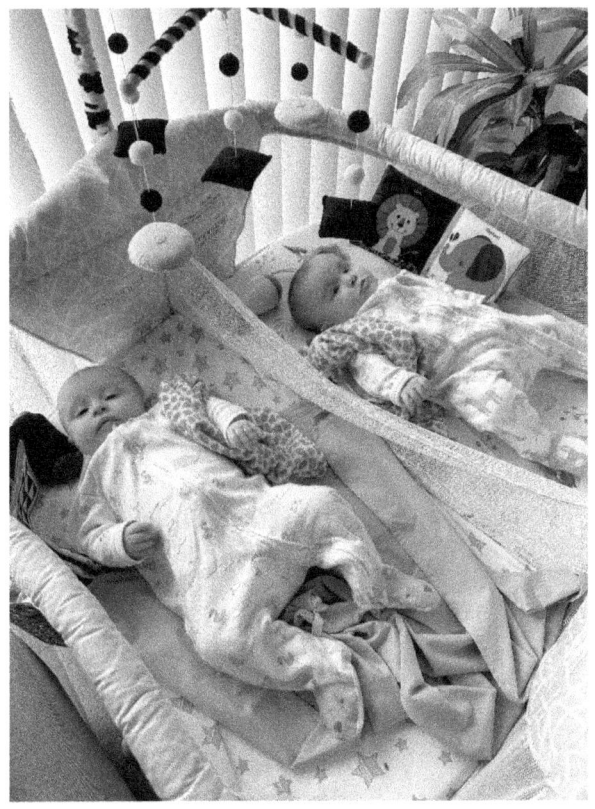

Rocking Chairs

You will probably need a rocking chair or a comfy place to sit. We purchased two chairs called "Gliders," one downstairs in our living room, and another for the twin's nursery. They are basically rocking chairs that doubled as recliners, which was so amazing. These chairs are one of the best purchases we have ever made. Not only was it great for holding babies and rocking them to sleep, it was also great for taking short naps in them once we could put the twins down in their bassinets. As I am writing this book, it has been almost two years, and we still use these gliders every day.

Cribs

It will be important to purchase separate cribs for your babies for their nursery, but it may not be used for 4-6 months. We had the cribs purchased and set up prior to the twins arrival, but it was used for extra storage those first few months with stockpiles of diapers and wipes. They now both sleep in their own cribs next to each other every night.

Dresser / Changing Table

We opted for a dresser where we could put a changing table on top of it to save space within our nursery. Some people choose to have a separate changing table in addition to their dresser, but that is your personal preference. We had a small pack n play changing table downstairs, which we used during the first few months, but we have found having a changing table on top of the dresser in the nursery, as they have grown bigger, to be a huge help. Though it is nice to separate all the onesies and clothing into a dresser, this may not be used as much as you may think in the first few months. As they start wearing more outfits down the road, you can separate the clothes in the drawers, but just note that during the first few months, they typically wore footed pajamas.

The next two items are not furniture, but are worth purchasing. The first is an LED baby light. The little night lights will help when you want to have some light in the room, but your normal house light is too bright for the babies while they sleep. Some look like eggs and others look like cylinders. We purchased two different kinds since we wanted one in two different rooms, but wanted to try different options to see which we liked more. Both kinds of lights have dimming functions for your liking. The better of the two, which we found, has not only a night light function, but it can also play ambient sounds like white noise or running water. It has an app which allows you to control the volume, the sounds, the color of the light, and how bright or dim you want it.

The second device I would suggest would be a noise shusher. It is a small speaker that makes the shushing sound which is so comforting to the baby, but also saves your voice along the way. This shusher helped us out so much when a baby started to wiggle around, almost waking up. The moment we turned the device on, the babies would fall back to sleep (most of the time).

What do you not need yet? Baby proofing items! Unless you have older children already, this is something which you should not need to worry about adding baby locks on your drawers or cabinets. Since they won't be crawling or walking for a while, you will have plenty of time to take care of all of this later.

You won't need to worry about baby proofing the house yet until they start crawling and walking. You will have a lot of time before that happens and have more important things to worry about when you come home.

I feel like there are a ton of different baby items that you might consider purchasing prior to the twins' arrival in addition to the required furniture. Sometimes putting brand names in books like this can be a little bit of a grey area, so I won't go into details of what specific brand names we used; however, there are many options based on your preferences for these items. These are some of the must-have items which we couldn't live without, especially when setting the house up for the babies.

Diaper Pail

Though there are many different brands out there, these pails are seriously the best for dirty diapers. I found that they were definitely worth the money to ensure that the house doesn't smell like diapers all the time.. Let's be real here, you will use A LOT of diapers with your twins. I actually had bought two of these, one for upstairs and downstairs so that I didn't have to worry about transporting the diapers up and down the stairs. It has been a huge lifesaver.

Diapers

I suggest you do a diaper raffle at the MOM's baby shower to start collecting diapers for your twins. It's a simple way to get different sizes right at the start. Diapers come in different sizes (Preemie, Newborn, #1, #2, #3, etc). Each size diaper indicates the weight and size of your baby. As your baby grows, they will move up in diaper size. You may find that sometimes one of your babies will be in a bigger size than the other. It may be important to buy two different sizes to ensure you have it available just in case. We like to bulk buy our diapers and buy from warehouse stores to save money! You may find a more preferred diaper brand you like more; however, if people want to give you diapers, **never** decline this offer. You are going to go through a lot of diapers, and every pack of diapers is going to help!

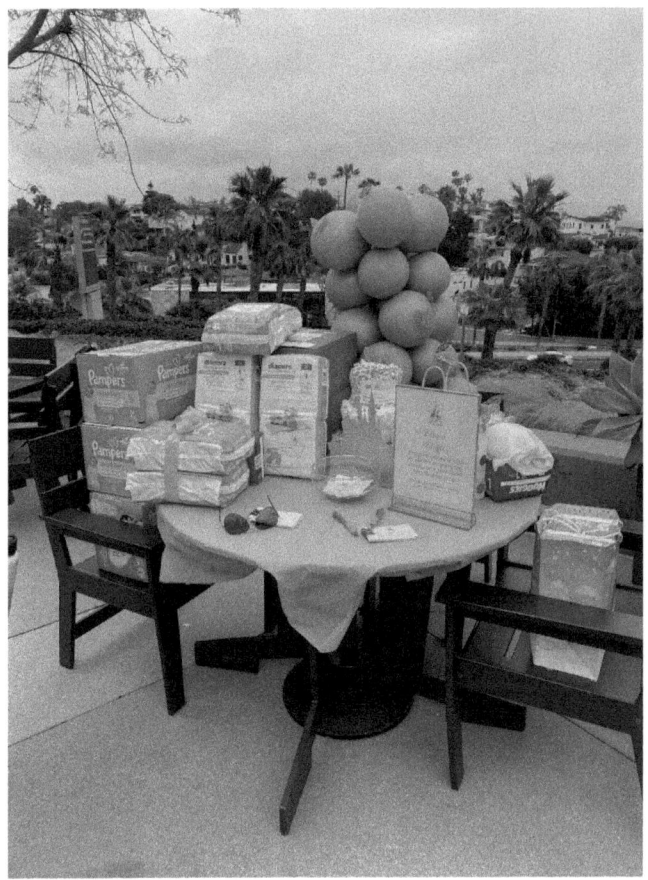

Baby Wipes

Let me tell you, it's going to be A LOT of baby wipes. Though some wipes are better or healthier than others, some companies have water wipes, which do not have any chemicals in them. If you can, I suggest you purchase these wipes in bulk! It's important to have these handy anywhere your baby might be (downstairs, upstairs, the car, diaper bag, etc.) because you never know when your babies might leave you little surprises. If you can buy these in bulk, you should! You will use all of them, trust me.

I know I went into how to wipe your baby depending on their gender in Chapter 6, but something to add here is the correct way to wipe and place a new diaper under the old diaper. In order to limit the amount of stress on your baby's spine, you should roll your baby on the side to wipe their butt to make sure you get all the excess poop. The old way that was more common was to lift up both of their legs straight up. This has since been found to cause back problems down the road.

We personally did not use a baby wipe warmer. The NICU did not use them, and we were told by a friend that their warmer caused an infection on their baby's private parts because of a fungus that grew within the warm environment of the warmer. They had to clean the warmer with bleach each time they changed out the pack of wipes. We never had any issues with not using a warmer. It sometimes made the babies wiggle more because the wipe was colder; however, the preference is up to you whether you decide to purchase a warmer.

Onesies and Clothing

As you invest in clothing for your little ones, you should ALWAYS buy the onesie options with zippers! From my experience, buttons and snaps are the worst when the snaps get stuck at 2 in the morning. If you can find footed onesies which have 2 zippers that you can unzip from both the top and the bottom, I found that those were so much easier to use to change diapers and still help to keep your baby still warm from the waist up.

Bottles

Though there are many different types of brands out there, I recommend finding an anti-colic style of bottles. These bottles help the babies not to consume as much air while feeding, which also helps to decrease spit-ups, helps with burping, and reduces colic. Our NICU nurses suggested we use a certain brand of bottles during our time there, and we just continued using those bottles once we came home, though we had another brand that was gifted to us at the baby shower. We found that they worked really well. They have both a narrow nipple and a wide nipple option for their bottle. If your baby is breastfeeding, the wide-neck bottles are the most similar to a real nipple, so this can help transition them to a bottle more easily. We actually use both personally, one type for each twin. Not only did it make it easier not to mix up the bottles, but the twins actually prefer the different ones. We had a problem with one of the twins' mouths getting burned from the nanny we hired. She warmed up the milk too hot, which caused one baby to have a more sensitive response to the bottle, so after consulting with medical staff, she ended up transitioning her to the wide mouth bottles since that was the only way to get her to drink milk during her recovery time. She ultimately just-preferred to have the wide nipple bottle after all was said and done. We decided that having multiple types of bottles was okay because, ultimately, whatever it took for her to drink her milk was the most important. My only complaint with the brand of bottle we used was how many parts there were to clean. Cleaning them thoroughly can be a little time-consuming due to the small areas around the parts.

Baby Bottle Warmers

We liked one brand so much that we used their products not only for the bottle warmer, but also for the next couple of products on this list. A bottle warmer is super helpful since microwaving milk can be dangerous and can cause the milk to be unevenly heated, which can ultimately burn your baby's mouth. Also, if you are pumping, heating up breast milk in the microwave can actually destroy some of the key nutrients. We liked that we could set the warmer to the appropriate amount of ounces we needed heated, and whether we were heating it from room temperature or cold. Our warmer would beep once the time ran out for the perfect warmth for the bottle. Obviously, you need to do the temperature test on your wrist to make sure it is okay first. There are lots of brands out there for warmers, I recommend you do some research on which one you like. Some have extra bells and whistles that help you out.

Baby Bottle Sterilizer and Dryer

Having one of these was highly suggested by pediatricians to sterilize the bottles in between uses. This helps prevent bacteria growth within the bottles from all the milk. There are different options which include counter top ones and microwave bags. Some people have found using a dishwasher works in the same way; however, the choice is up to you.

Formula Dispenser

Since our twins were in the NICU, they came home on a higher caloric formula intake, which required us to make their milk the old-fashioned way by boiling the water and adding the formula at a certain temperature, which was suggested by the formula manufacturers because the formula itself is not sterile. So, when you follow the instructions on the label, it is supposed to help kill any added bacteria in the formula. We made the formula this way for about 3 months, and then we switched to a formula dispenser when we were given the go-ahead to the normal measurements. This was perhaps the best decision we ever made. This device automatically dispenses the formula powder and warm water all in about 5 seconds. There was no more boiling and refrigerating anymore, and that was a major win and time saver.

Baby Monitors

Though there are so many different types of baby monitors around, you should definitely find one that has a great picture and sound quality. You should also look for a monitor that has night vision and sound monitoring, as well as zoom capability, and even shows room temperature. We chose to opt for a camera that was not WiFi connected to ensure no one else could connect to our cameras to watch the twins; however, there are multiple cameras out on the market where you can connect to your home WiFi and watch the camera remotely through your phone. It really depends on your specific wants and needs. We just chose to have security over ease.

Baby Monitoring Socks

We used a big brand name for these, but there are other great ones on the market. These socks monitor your baby's heart rate and blood oxygen levels, especially when they go to sleep. Coming out of the NICU, we were used to hearing alarms that would trigger if there was any drop in our baby's heart rate or oxygen levels, which adds anxiety to your little ones coming home. These socks truly gave us peace of mind at night to know that we would be alerted if something were to happen. Though not every parent likes to use these since they can be a little temperamental and can have false alarms due to the baby not in range of the base station, or even a loss of Bluetooth connection. The choice is ultimately up to you; however, it helped us tremendously and gave us improved sleep (though being a twin parent, sleep is difficult to come by in the first few months).

The last point I will add here for setting up the house for the babies isn't something to buy, but the House and Room Temperature - At this point, writing the book, the current medical temperature recommendation for babies to be in is 68-72 degrees Fahrenheit (20-22 degrees Celsius). This is found to be the optimal range for babies and to prevent SIDS (Sudden Infant Death Syndrome). There are multiple reasons that cause SIDS, and a warm room temperature is one of them. For this reason, pediatricians will recommend these cooler temperature ranges in the house for babies.

Chapter Four: Setting up for You and Your Wife

Setting you and your wife up for success will greatly help in the beginning. Anything to make your lives easier and streamlined will be of major benefit. Once you streamline normal daily life, you are able to focus more on your babies to help meet all of their needs.

In the first few weeks that you come home, the thought of leaving the house will seem daunting. There will be very little sleep, so planning ahead of time is necessary. The first thing to have a plan for is groceries, including snacks. Buying in bulk, if you are able to, is helpful, as you may not get out of the house as much as you are used to once your babies arrive. I suggest you try to buy products that are as healthy as you can because when you first bring your babies home, you will not be sleeping very much. You don't want to feed your body junk food and then feel even worse than you will or get sick. Products like mixed nuts and sugar-free protein bars were some of our favorite snacks to have available on our living room table for easy snacking when we chose to do contact napping with our twins.

For main meals, I would suggest food prepping ahead of time. Cooking multiple meals at a time and freezing will be such a time saver when you are juggling feeding and changing diapers. This can also include breakfasts. I personally liked to make scrambled eggs with mixed vegetables, cheese, and sour cream. I also used to make hard-boiled eggs in big batches because the eggs last a few days in the fridge. This was a lifesaver for us when we wanted a snack at 2 in the morning, but didn't want to have a big meal. We bought an automatic hard-boiled egg maker, and it was such a good purchase at the time, and we definitely got our money's worth out of it.

I also had a reach-in freezer, so I was able to cook and prepare meals for 2-3 weeks at a time and freeze them. It made it super simple because we just needed to defrost the meal in the microwave, and it was ready to eat. For meals, we ate a lot of meat and veggies and all sorts of tacos/ fajitas, etc. You may think that this will be repetitive; however, you don't have to stay plain and bland here. There are so many different types of sauces, rubs, veggies, meats, and flavors to keep you going during this time.

The next thing you should focus on streamlining is house chores and cleaning. Cleaning every day is so tiring, especially when you have to wash double sets of bottles, but having a set time of the day you do things helps keep everything on track. One of the super handy tricks that helped us keep the dishes down was to use paper plates and plastic cups. Keeping up with the laundry, completing your chores, and getting ready every day will also help you mentally. It's never fun to trip over old clothing or knock over a cup that's left over from 3 days ago.

If you're using it, buying formula in bulk will be helpful too. This goes for formula water, diapers, and wipes. Buying from big box stores or online helps with extra savings. Let me tell you every penny saved will be key when you are buying double of everything for twins!.

Chapter Five: Closer to Birth

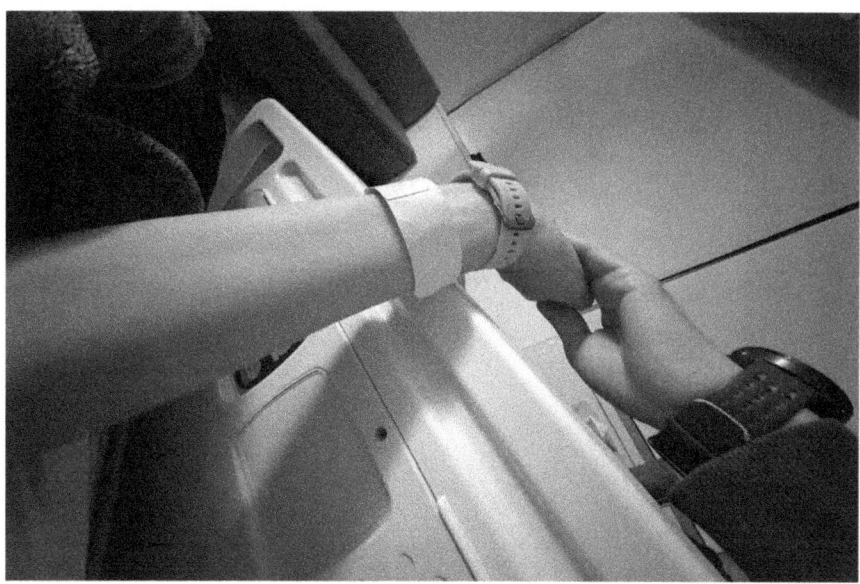

As the time gets closer, the doctors will ask you if MOM would like to deliver the twins naturally or via C-Section(cesarean section). We were told the safest procedure for everyone involved with multiples is the C-Section. If MOM is able to get closer to the full term for a twin pregnancy at 36.5 weeks, then natural is an option. However, if something happens during the pregnancy, then the obvious choice is to have a C-Section to remove the babies before full term. The doctors typically will not allow the babies to go to the 40-week mark, which is full term for a singleton, because it just gets too crowded in MOM's tummy and can cause more harm than good.

At this point in the book, we have already discussed about MOM going to a high risk doctor. They will watch MOM and the babies to ensure everything is going well. However, if something is not perfect, the doctors will run tests and have MOM do things to help the babies. This includes things like bed rest, coming into their office more often for ultrasounds, or even spending time in the hospital under 24 hour nursing care.

Antepartum

If the doctors send MOM to the hospital earlier than expected, she will probably end up on the Antepartum floor. This literally means "before birth." My wife spent 7 weeks in the hospital under Antepartum care; however, most women won't require this long of a stay. We had certain circumstances that required her to stay in the hospital and not send her back home.

If MOM arrives at this Antepartum section, chances are the babies are coming soon. MOM gets sent to the hospital for many reasons, including abnormal heartbeats, poor umbilical cord flow, stunted growth, Preeclampsia (Mom's high blood pressure), or even MOM's high blood sugar. Both MOM and the babies will be under 24/7 watch.

As soon as you get to the room, the doctors and nurses are constantly in and out, introducing themselves, running tests, starting MOM's arm IV, and giving you information on what is happening. Social workers and NICU doctors will also visit and introduce themselves. They will provide information about what their hospital section is and what to expect from them. Try to keep up, or even take notes on your phone, so you can refer back to them. It can be overwhelming; taking notes allows you to go back and digest the information when you exit the room and helps formulate questions for your doctor should any arise.

Though this can be done at a normal lab setting, if you are sent to the hospital between 24-28 weeks, the nurses will do a blood sugar test. This Glucose Challenge Test (GCT) is a screening test where you drink a sugary drink, and your blood sugar is measured one hour later and three hours later. This is to check if MOM has Gestational Diabetes. If MOM fails this test, then the nursing staff will go over the remedies and options for you. Detecting if MOM has Gestational Diabetes is important because it can lead to complications for both the mother and baby, including high blood pressure, large babies, and increased risk of type 2 diabetes later in life.

If you are sent to the hospital early for any reason, there may be a chance that they will inform you that MOM should get a round of steroid shots (betamethasone). These steroids are designed to help strengthen the babies' lungs a little bit more if they are to be delivered early. The MOM would be required to get two injections during a 24-hour time frame. My wife and I agreed to these shots because we wanted to do anything that would possibly help the babies have a good delivery and a chance of life after. Like I said before, though, it is always your choice for any procedure

As part of being monitored within the antepartum section, the nurses will run many NSTs (Non-Stress Test) for the MOM and the babies. It is a prenatal test that monitors the baby's heart rate and movements to assess fetal well-being. Don't worry, it is not invasive, and it looks like a little disk that the nurses place on MOM's belly to listen to the babies and differentiate the MOMs heartbeat as well. If they determine that one of these tests does not give them good results within the 20-40 minute time frame and a baby is in trouble in the womb, this would call for an immediate delivery. Keep in mind, your babies might like to move and can "fall off the monitor." This may require additional time to be monitored during the NST. Our Baby B was notorious for wiggling around when it was time to complete the NST, which made it seem that her heart rate dropped off. Finally, one of the nurses was able to tie down the monitor on my wife's stomach with extra straps and a washcloth just to ensure they were able to get a good read for the required length of time.

Nurses leap into action, and sometimes it may not be what you need or want. For instance, one of the night nurses came into my wife's room to give her a shot of some type of medication; however, my wife was not supposed to receive this shot, nor did she want it. After stopping and questioning the nurse about it, the nurse realized she was in the wrong room and it was supposed to go to a different patient. We don't know what the shot was or what would have happened if we weren't on guard. This isn't to scare you, but accidents can happen, so you have to stay vigilant and alert.

Chapter Six: Hospital and Delivery

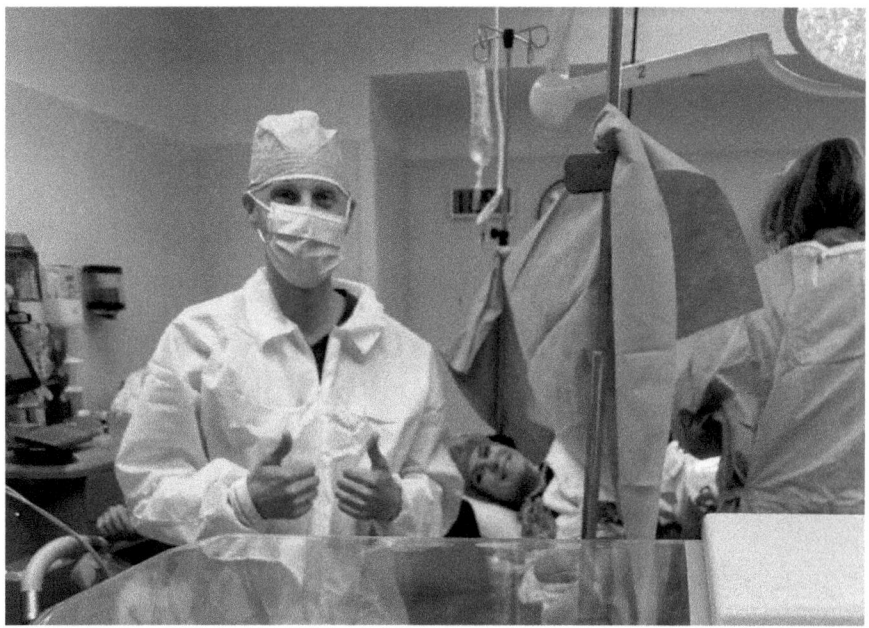

What to pack for your hospital stay

You will need two "go bags." One for you and one for MOM.

DAD's go bag is pretty easy. Toiletries and a change of clothes, things to be comfortable in the hospital and something you are okay with taking pictures in. I also recommend having a button up shirt so that you have the ability to do skin to skin contact with the babies easier. Also having some snacks packed will save you since you may not always have the opportunity to go to the cafeteria at certain times of the day.

MOM's go bag is the same with the addition of a few things. Ensure she packs some slippers and some clothes which are easy to get in and out of. Breastfeeding dresses or ones that unbutton on her shoulders are a great option, especially if she is breastfeeding or pumping. She will be in a lot of pain following delivery and possibly drugged up a little bit so ease of use is best here.

Some non-essential options to pack, which we loved having in our hospital room, were a Bluetooth speaker, to listen to music prior to and after delivery. We also had multiple 10 ft. charging cables for our phones because not all rooms have electrical outlets near the beds and couch areas. We also ended up packing the Amazon TV stick so that my wife could watch her favorite shows on the TV, versus having to watch the boring hospital-selected channels and movies.

Though every hospital is different, some rooms are very cold. Having a thicker blanket or a comforter to use while you stay on the pull-out couch is a must as the DAD. You can always have MOM ask the nurses for a warm blanket and/ or a foam mattress pad to lie down on the pull-ut couch, and that is a game changer too! Comfort for DAD is also important! This one was a little funny for us. My wife asked for an extra bed foam pad for "her" so I could use it. The hospital is not a hotel, and they typically do not want to accommodate any extra people. My wife was able to sweet-talk a night nurse to leave the extra foam pad in her room for when I stayed over. Since she was in the Antepartum section in the hospital for 7 weeks, I used that foam pad quite a bit to help pad that terribly uncomfortable couch.

Delivery

Delivery is a big one, the main event!!

The Ultimate Twin Dad Survival Guide

As you come to the hospital, the nurses and doctors will kick into gear and do what they need to do for MOM and babies. Now, unless something is going wrong with MOM or the babies, the nurses do their best to keep everyone calm by blocking you from seeing their setup activities. If something is happening and the babies require an emergency C-section, the staff will still be calm, but everything moves a lot faster. I witnessed this firsthand with my wife's delivery.

My wife had some type of blood pressure issue where if she was lying just right and a blanket was on her legs, she would overheat and get dizzy, and her blood pressure would drop. This was somehow caused by the pregnancy or the umbilical cord locations, but no one could figure out what was the real cause. It happened a few times when she was getting ultrasounds and freaked the nurses out there. However, on the day of delivery, if this happens, it calls for an immediate emergency. While prepping for the C-Section, a nurse had placed a heated blanket over my wife to keep her warm after she was given the spinal tap. Not realizing the magnitude of the heated blanket on her and her past issues, after only a minute had passed, she started overheating, and her blood pressure dropped, and so did the baby's heart rate. Since this happened in the Operating Room, the doctor who was attending to her called an emergency, and all of the nurses and doctors came rushing in. I was just sitting in the waiting section playing on my phone when the door swung open and over 10 people came out saying it's go time. When I got into the room, my wife filled me in on what had happened. I knew that they were thinking the babies were in trouble and they needed to be delivered. My wife and I said that there was no point in bringing up the past issues with the blankets to all the doctors and operating room staff because there was no point as everything was already in motion. Once the procedure started, the babies were both out in roughly 3 minutes.

Timeline of what you should expect should you require a C-Section

You will arrive at the hospital and check in.

You will be taken to a staging room / prep area. You may be in this staging area with multiple families. They will at least have the area you are in curtained off for some privacy. MOM will lie down in a hospital bed to have multiple IVs inserted into her arm. It will be one IV for her, and one IV for each baby she is carrying. They will also set MOM up to have an NST to monitor the baby's heart beats prior to entering the operating room. There will be one monitor for each baby and one for the mother's heartbeat, which can be on her belly or a finger pulse Oximeter to keep track of her blood oxygen levels.

The doctors and the nurses will stop by and introduce themselves, take medical history, and will review any special delivery requests / birth plan you may have prepared. Be prepared to answer a lot of questions, but they will also give you a rundown of what will happen next as things move forward.

After all the prep has been completed, MOM will then be taken into the delivery room. She will be prepped for surgery. If applicable, the anesthesiologist will be in the room with the nurses and will administer the spinal tap. This is where they use a local anesthetic to numb the lower back before a needle is inserted to extract spinal fluid.

During this time, the nurses prepare the surgery room for the big moment.

The best way I can describe this next part is controlled chaos. There are a lot of doctors and nurses moving to get your babies out safely. There will be a team of doctors for MOM, and then each baby will have their own team of doctors and nurses which are looking out for them. It is quite chaotic, but everyone is doing what they are supposed to do.

They will offer to you and MOM to see what is happening during the C-Section with a mirror, or you can request a transparent sheet to watch during the surgery. My wife and I opted for the "No Thank You" response to this. Some people want to see the babies coming out, but I am not sure I would have stayed conscious if I had seen it.

At this point, I will warn you that if MOM goes through a C-Section, they are a little brutal. I guess normal labor is tough as well, but with a C-Section, they are tugging back and forth on MOM. It was hard for me to be in the room and witness it as a caring husband who had to see my wife go through it. The two amazing babies that came from it were worth it, though.

During the delivery, you will be able to take pictures or video. DAD will usually be offered to trim the umbilical cords. I personally declined doing this because I did not want to see any of my wife's surgery and the blood. I wasn't sure if I would freak out or faint, so I opted out of that one.

Once the babies are born and the umbilical cords have been cut, the doctors may need to take them to the Neonatal ICU (NICU) for additional monitoring. This means that MOM will not be able to do the skin-to-skin contact that she may have envisioned. For reference, both of our babies were in an isolette wrapped in plastic to maintain their heat and wheeled directly to the NICU as soon as they were stable. As the dad, you will usually be asked to follow them, as the other doctors take care of MOM and continue to stitch or staple the wound opening. In the NICU, the doctors will explain the situation for each of the babies and provide you with a rundown of what they will do next.

Once MOM gets stitched/stapled back up, they will take her back to the recovery room to keep an eye on her for a while. She will be on her own during this time, which will be difficult for her since both you and her babies will be in another part of the hospital. You will be able to go back and visit her at this point. Reassure her and remind her how amazing she is for bringing those miracles into the world, and support her during this time. Since she will be coming off the anesthesia, she will be shaking quite a bit. This is completely normal as they wear off, but may seem unsettling to see.

After the recovery room, MOM will go up to the postpartum hospital room. This will be your home away from home for approximately 3-4 days for recovery. During this time, the nurses and doctors will teach MOM about milk production, collection, and how to support your babies when they come home. They will also be checking on the wound status to ensure there is no infection or concerns prior to leaving the hospital. You will have plenty of time here to ask as many questions as you can. Also, I would recommend obtaining the phone numbers of any extra resources they offer. These might come in handy if you have any more questions once the babies come home. Trust me, there are lots of questions.

From here, the recovery at home for MOM takes a couple of weeks. You will need to help your wife with walking up the stairs, trips to the bathroom, taking a shower, driving her places, or back to the hospital if your babies need continued NICU stay time, etc. Her body just went through a major trauma, and she needs your help and compassion. This is your chance to be the awesome husband I know you are.

Timeline of what you should expect should you require a Natural Birth.

1. The timeline for a natural birth is almost the same, but with a few different details, obviously. MOM will wear the fetal monitoring equipment for both babies because natural birth for multiples has an increased risk of complications. The labor process is basically the same as a singleton, but with a second pushing stage for the second baby. Usually delivered within 10-30 minutes of each other.

2. Once the first baby is delivered, it is handed off to the first NICU team for evaluation, and attention is then turned to the second twin.

3. An ultrasound will be performed to check the position of the second twin. If the second twin is in a good (head down) position, then things will proceed as normal. If the second twin is facing breach (butt down) then this can be a problem and the doctors will try to move the baby around to face the other way. However, if they are

unsuccessful, there will most likely be a C-Section for the safety of the baby.

4. Once the second twin is born, they are also handed off to the NICU team for evaluation.

5. The doctors will fill you in as time goes, explaining what they are doing and what to expect.

6. During the delivery, you will be able to take pictures or video. DAD will usually be offered to trim the umbilical cords. This is optional, and some fathers decide they want to be involved within the delivery process. There will be medical professionals available to cut the cord should you choose to opt out..

7. MOM's recovery will be slightly different if everything is natural, but she will still need a lot of help with the day-to-day tasks for a couple of weeks. Be sure to help out while she is recovering. You being there for her during those next weeks will mean more to her than you know. Surprise her with her favorite meal that she hasn't had when she was pregnant, or bring her a bouquet of flowers. Little gestures go a long way, after all, she has carried your babies for the last 9 months.

Chapter Seven: Babies' First Moments

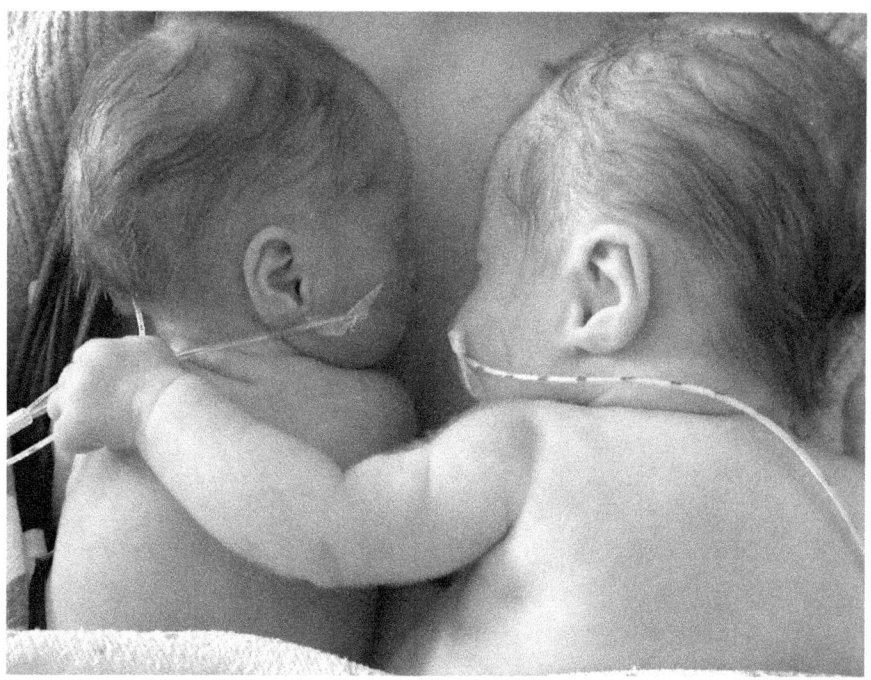

There is a dedicated team of doctors and nurses just for each individual baby. Once the baby is born, the team leaps into action, and each person has their own tasks to perform. They make sure everything is going well with the health of your baby. If something is not right, they should catch it here and provide the baby with some extra care.

The doctors will perform an APGAR assessment and give your babies a score at 1 and 5 minutes after birth. An APGAR score is a standardized assessment of the baby's status immediately after birth and the response to resuscitation efforts. It stands for Appearance (Skin Color), Pulse (Heart Rate), Grimace Response (Reflexes),

Activity (Muscle Tone), and Respiration (Breathing Rate and Effort). The first score at the one-minute mark evaluates how well your newborn tolerated the birth process, and the score at the five-minutes will tell how your baby is transitioning to life. Each section gets a score of 0-2 and will all get added up from 0-10 for the total score. A score of 7 or above means your baby is in good health. A lower score does not necessarily mean they have bad health; it mainly means they will need more immediate medical care. These scores help the medical staff make decisions about if the baby needs more or less medical care right away. As an example, my personal first score was a 2/10, and my second score was 5/10. This helped the staff determine how to help me out after the complications with my delivery.

The overall health and weight of the babies will determine what happens next. If they are very small, they may be placed in a plastic bag to help hold in the heat (head outside of the bag of course). They will be placed into the Isolette before they are taken to the NICU if needed. Many preterm babies need to spend some time in the NICU. More information on that is in the next section. If your babies are healthy enough, the doctors will most likely ask if you want to do skin-to-skin contact. This is crucial for the babies. Do this skin-to-skin if you are able to.

One of the most amazing sounds in the world was hearing our babies cry for the first time as they breathed air for the first time. Even though we weren't able to hold them, this sound gave both my wife and me so much joy. Just know that even if you don't hear their cry right away, you shouldn't worry too much at the beginning, especially since some babies may need more time or attention. It sounds cliche, but that first cry from your little babies will be one you will always remember.

Over the next 24 hours, you can expect a few things in the hospital. Some babies are able to feed within the first few hours, making a good opportunity to start trying to breastfeed. But a lot of the time, the babies will be tired and need to sleep. The nurses and doctors will come into your room and will help MOM set up her breast pump and assist with initial production. If the hospital allows the MOM to rent out a hospital-grade breast pump, I would highly recommend it. When you have multiples or even preterm babies, these pumps help MOM's initial supply to be established. Our hospital allowed us to bring one of these pumps home for a couple of weeks until we could obtain ours through insurance.

In most hospitals, the baby's first bath will be done right in the hospital recovery room. This is the chance for the staff to go over bathing instructions for you. Water temps, type of soaps, and baby holding techniques are very important. The nurses will also go over how to do diaper changes at this point and correct wiping. For boys, there is no specific requirement, so either way, wiping up or down is fine. For girls, you are required to wipe their area from top to bottom, wiping front to back. This wiping technique for the girls is crucial because you don't want to cause any infections by wiping in the incorrect direction.

If your babies are healthy enough to go home with you at this point, the nurses will do a final physical before you leave. They will check for malformations, look for any signs of infection, look for any signs of jaundice, and monitor breathing. Additionally, they will also listen for heart murmurs, check to make sure babies' bowls are functioning properly, and check for any unnatural soft spots on the head. The nurses may also take a small blood sample to check for any metabolic diseases that would be good to know about as early as possible.

Before checking out of the hospital, be aware that a social worker will most likely stop by to check on MOM's emotional state. They want to make sure they address any changes in her mental state prior to releasing the baby to your care. If there is any concern or additional questions, ensure the MOM utilizes this time with the medical staff. They are there to help in any way they can.

Chapter Eight: NICU Time

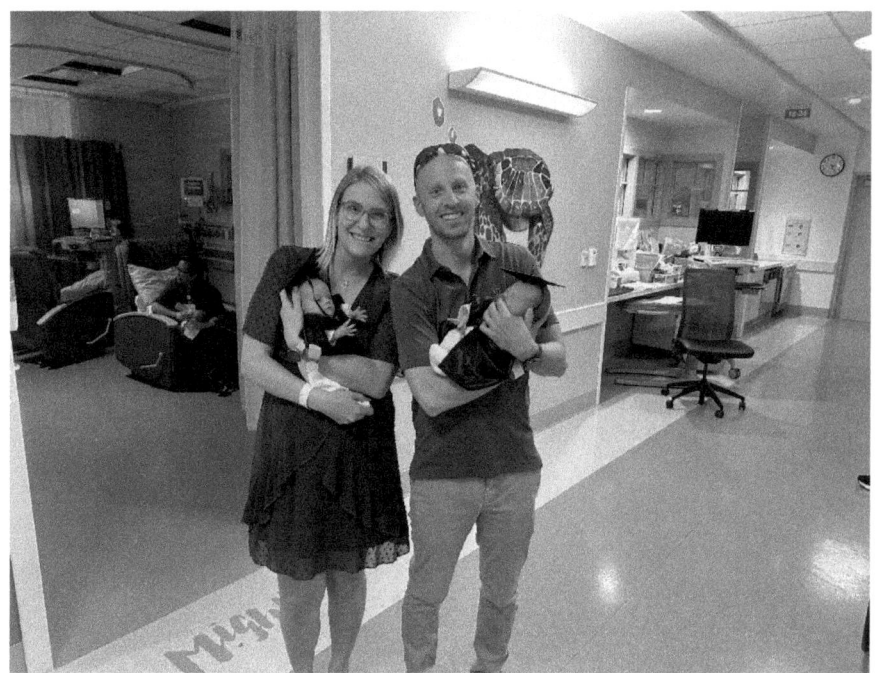

Disclaimer: This chapter really focuses on required NICU (Neonatal Intensive Care Unit) time; however, not every set of twins require a NICU stay, but many do so I wanted to make sure I addressed some of the topics here.

If your twins require time within the NICU, you will probably already know at the point of delivery. The doctors say a good rule of thumb is that babies usually stay in the hospital until right around their 40-week due date if they deliver early. All babies born before 28 weeks are categorized as "extremely premature," and those born before 37 weeks of pregnancy are categorized as "premature." Because of this, each of these babies was born too early for their organs to fully develop, which can also lead to health problems. With time and care, most premature babies grow to become healthy kids with no problems at all. So, take a deep breath and understand that even though this might be a stressful time, the medical staff are the most equipped to assist your little one.

Though you might have gone directly from the operating room to the NICU when one or both of your babies were born, the doctors and nurses will wheel the MOM up to see the babies. Though at the time, she might not have a skin-to-skin contact opportunity, this is the time you will be able to hold their fingers for the first time and take more pictures of your little ones. There will be more opportunities throughout the first few days in the hospital to take a wheelchair to the NICU to see your little ones.

In the NICU, the nurses and doctors have their own vocabulary that can seem overwhelming at times. It's important to ask questions and definitions if you don't understand what they mean. I was always asking questions each day. To really start grasping all of the information, it's important to show up each morning during the daily doctor's morning rounds. This is when the doctor on call goes to each baby's bedside and each on-duty nurse provides the doctor the most recent, up- to-date information about the baby's health and how the previous day and night shift went. The doctor will then provide instructions for the day of what changes they want to see or if they want to keep things status quo. This goes from adjusting oxygen flow, increasing food amounts, adjusting any medicine, etc. Being present for these rounds was so helpful to understand what is going on. They even give you a chance to ask any questions about what you heard and how your babies are doing. There may be times when you think the doctor's suggestion is taking a step back from the progress your little one has made, but keep in mind the ultimate goal is to make sure your baby is healthy enough to come home.

The babies may initially start with lots of tubes and monitoring equipment on them. You can ask what each piece of equipment is for. As they grow, the nurses and doctors will slowly take away the extra equipment which is no longer needed. Make sure to celebrate the small victories like this, if the hospital does not provide a journal, I recommend you having a small notepad where you can write down information along the way from their daily weights, to any changes in their health, to even these small victories. The time your little ones stay in the NICU can be overwhelming and you may forget what happened a week before or even a day before. This journal is a great reference tool that you can look back to during your stay.

You will also be offered to have skin to skin holding time. It may not be on the first day or even the second day; however, when the opportunity arise, do this as much as you can as it helps regulate your baby's vitals like heart rate and temperature, stimulates breast feeding, and can significantly reduce stress in the newborns as they try to adapt to life outside of the womb. It also promotes bonding between the parent and newborn and can help reduce postpartum depression in mothers.

When you enter the NICU, it may not be the quiet nursery you might have anticipated. There are many alarms that go off for each baby and each monitor which is attached to them. Though some alarms are okay, and some are not. At the beginning you might worry a little bit with each one so remember to ask questions. After a while you'll think to yourself, "Oh, feeding time is over" when you hear a certain tone. The nurses know what all of the alarms are and will leap into action if needed. It can be stressful for the parent to watch their baby need a little bit of help or extra stimulation to breathe, but just try to remember that they are in the NICU to receive that much needed help.

Be prepared for the doctors and nurses to offer and even push vaccines for your babies. This is ALWAYS your choice. They may make you feel bad or worried if you decline. Hepatitis B is pushed to be given to your babies before you leave the hospital because studies show that if they are able to get you to give your kids a vaccine early on, you will continue the vaccination schedule later. You and MOM will probably be tested prior to delivery, so you will already know if the babies will have it at birth. Hepatitis B is typically only passed via needles and drug use, or through sex workers as an STD. It is what is called a blood borne pathogen. I'm not trying to sway you either way, but this is the information that the doctors will not tell you. They have rules of what they can and cannot tell you per their hospital policy. But remember, hospitals are businesses that are there to make money. I will talk a little more about vaccines in Chapter 12.

When it comes closer for your babies to come home, the doctors will require the name of your pediatrician which your babies will be going to. This is to ensure your babies continue to get healthcare when they are discharged. I suggest finding someone in your area and conduct a small interview ahead of time to see if you are comfortable with one and choose accordingly. My wife and I interviewed four different pediatricians prior to the girls being born. We found the perfect one for us that aligned with our wants and needs. She was even a twin mom herself which has also helped a ton for twin related questions.

The final note I will mention about the NICU is the tests the babies need to pass prior to your little one's discharge. The babies need to have a certain amount of days since their last event where they needed help from a nurse to breathe or have any heart rate problems. The next test is the car seat test. The nurses will place your baby in a car seat with all of their monitors attached. This test should be completed in the same car seat you will use to bring your baby home. This test will last for one hour and will require them not to have any drop in their blood oxygen level during that time. This is to ensure that they will be able to safely make it home without any problems. One of our twins took a couple of tries to pass. Another side note is that your baby will need to be a certain weight to safely fit in the car seat. So even if your baby passes all the required tests, if they are not at the required weight to use the car seat, they will not be allowed to be discharged. There is also a requirement to be able to take enough food without a feeding tube. The babies need to be able to drink enough milk that they will get enough calories to be sent home. Just note that if the MOM is also breastfeeding, the NICU staff takes that into account during this time. However, there is a small possibility that if they meet all of the other tests, but still struggle with this, at some point the doctors may discharge the baby with a feeding tube for you. I know of one couple that had to do this. It took maybe about two weeks after being sent home for the baby to be able to take enough milk to not use the tube anymore.

This time may seem like long days and can be stressful at times. For me, I knew it was more important for our babies to be in the NICU receiving 24 hour care than being home with us. It was hard leaving them there for the night, but some NICU locations have webcam availability where you could log in and see your baby after hours. It was nice to know you could still keep an eye on them, even if you weren't there.

When the day comes when your baby is discharged back home, make it a big celebration. They have come a long way since birth and it should be celebrated. We had a little graduation ceremony for each of the girls where we dressed them up in a cap and gown to celebrate their accomplishments. All the NICU nurses and doctors came and played pomp and circumstance and cheered their achievement. It was amazing to see everyone come together to root for the milestone your baby had achieved.

Chapter Nine: Coming Home from the Hospital

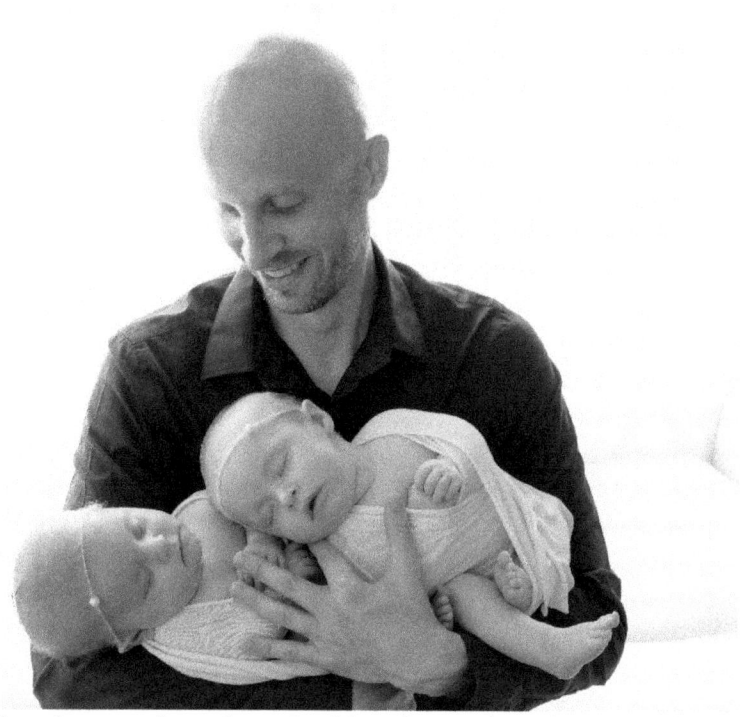

The day that you have been looking forward to since you found out you were going to be a dad has arrived. I have to say the first drive home with your baby/babies will be scary, especially if you did NICU time. Just note, it will all be okay. The biggest doctor suggestion is to not leave your baby in a car seat longer than the actual ride. The airway in their neck has not hardened yet like an adult, so their airway can get pinched if they sleep and relax too much in a car seat for too long. This is why the doctors do a car seat test before the babies are discharged, to make sure at least the drive home will be okay. Never let your baby nap in their car seat for this reason. I had my wife sit in the backseat with the babies to make sure there weren't any issues or breathing concerns. This just gave a little extra comfort to me since they were still so little.

Once home it will set in how difficult the beginning will be and nervous you will be. For us, the NICU alarms kind of scared us and we had a hard time adjusting to not being on high alert at all times. The lack of sleep, nerves, and crying will also take a toll on you.

I suggest getting a food delivery service, having a family member make you some food, or set up a meal train like i mentioned before. You don't want to have to cook while worrying about taking care of the babies. The first night we came home with both girls, a neighbor brought us our favorite meal, steak fajitas. As we pulled the car up they were walking out of the house to give us the food. We didn't ask for it, we didn't even tell them we were bringing the babies home that day. My wife and I knew that God had prompted them to help us out with a meal for the night. We were already stressed out over everything and there were some thankful tears from us that God was showing us some love.

That first night, one of our girls spit up and couldn't breathe until we turned her sideways and helped clear the spit up. The next day we called the pediatrician and asked what we could do to prevent that from happening again. She told us to hold the babies on a pillow with a little incline for about 20 minutes to help them digest all the milk prior to laying them down. This greatly helped with spit ups and colic.

The other suggestion the doctors at NICU and the pediatrician taught us about bottle feeding was what they call "sideline feeding." This is a type of feeding position that is being used more often especially with preterm babies who might have difficulties feeding. We would place the babies on their side on a pillow and facing their head towards the nipple which allowed us to control the flow of the bottle easier to prevent choking and reduced the air intake. It also made it a lot easier to burp the babies after feeding side line versus in the nook of your arm.

I have to say the real game changer with spit ups was when we were able to change to a better formula. I will dive into formulas a little more in the next chapter.

Chapter Ten: Formulas

You may or may not know by now, but breast milk is the best thing for your babies. It is natural and gives the babies what they need to grow. There are many studies showing the benefits of breast milk for babies. Unfortunately, not every mother is able to produce enough for both babies. This is where formula comes into play.

It's important to ALWAYS read the ingredient labels. Typical American big name brands use corn syrup, white sugar, and soybean oil. These brands clearly do not care about your baby's health, they only care about money. So as a parent it is so important to read the labels and buy better ingredient formulas. You may be asking why companies add these ingredients in something which we feed our babies with. The answer is mainly profit. If they are able to cut costs with ingredients they are able to make more money. Unfortunately, the health of our babies takes a back seat.

Companies have certain ingredients that by law they are required to add to baby formula. One of these ingredients sections is omega 6 fats. These fats are supposedly in breast milk so these companies are mandated by the government to be added in formula. Then enters in vegetable oils which are a good cheap source of these fats. Canola and soy are two main ones you'll typically see, but others tend to be mixed in as well. It is almost impossible to get away from them.

Another ingredient they cut corners with is carbohydrates. High fructose corn syrup solids and white sugar are cheap sources of carbohydrates. These are added even after the countless studies showing how bad they are for humans to consume, let alone babies. Unfortunately, they tend to be the option of choice since they are cheap and readily available.

Every formula company has to adhere to government regulations, which for most of the rest of the ingredients is a good thing. You want your baby to have all the necessary vitamins and nutrients they will need to grow well. Substituting formula for just plain milk would be detrimental to the health and wellness of your baby. Always follow your pediatrician's advice when it comes to timing of taking your baby off of formula to solid food or whole milk.

Some formula brands have good organic whole milk and lactose as the first ingredients. I actually bought formula online from Germany because of the cleaner ingredients. It was actually cheaper for us to import formulas, than purchasing the American brands. I am intentionally leaving out formula brand names here as you should buy what is best for you and your family. A simple online google search for organic baby formula should provide you a list of the latest offerings from around the world. Just make sure you read the ingredients lists and choose what is best for you with your pediatrician's approval.

Lactose intolerance in babies is an interesting topic. True lactose intolerance affects a very small percentage of babies. It's typically mis-diagnosed because the babies have a problem with a bad ingredient within the formula and lactose is immediately to blame. Sometimes the doctors or pediatrician will then suggest either a "plant based" soy formula, or a non-milk amino acid formula. If this is the case for you, remember you are the parent. Do your research and research more information yourself. If, after speaking with your pediatrician, you agree and determine a plant based formula is what you should do, find the best one with the most benefit. Just remember for the future, if you are a vegetarian, kids need good animal source protein and fats to grow well and be healthy. Some parents sacrifice the health of their children for an ideology. There will be plenty of time for them to make their own choice about their source of food later. I have family members that were raised and still are vegetarian and they've always had a lot of health problems, especially as they are getting into their 20s and 30s. These family members are paying the costs of their parents' actions. However to be fair, as they grow into adulthood, they now choose what they want to eat, but still choose vegetarianism. Regardless of the direction you decide, do what you have determined is best for your family.

Chapter Eleven: Pediatrician and What to Expect

The pediatrician visits are a place to ask new questions about your baby's health, nutrition, sleep habits, poops, anything you can think of! I suggest asking around with friends that share your views to see if they suggest any pediatrician in particular. We recommend you interview multiple doctors to find the one you like most, and you can always change later if you would like. You are not bound to the first pediatrician you choose. We found our pediatrician through getting a recommendation from someone in our church.

The pediatrician has two main purposes. The first purpose is to make sure your babies are growing, healthy, and you are being a responsible parent. The pediatrician is looking for signs of slow growth or malnutrition, along with good limber body movement. They will check for overall sickness and infections and prescribe any medication required or follow up therapy which may be required. They will also check to make sure you are being a good parent and are not hurting or abusing your baby in any way. Please don't ever be that type of person. I don't believe I need to say anything more here.

The second main purpose for a pediatrician is providing "vaccines." Since this is a very controversial subject, I'd like to state that this book has neither a Pro or Anti Vaccine stance and does not give medical advice. That is between you and your doctors. The point of this information is to provide you with some facts. Make your own decisions with MOM and your pediatrician according to your own family priorities.

Pediatricians are paid bonuses for vaccinating children. Major shot companies pay extra to have a certain percentage of patients getting the vaccines. For this reason, some pediatricians will no longer take children as patients should you refuse to give vaccines, and you will be required to find a new doctor.

If you look at data from 50 years ago to now and the vaccine schedule, there is a pretty clear correlation between the amount of vaccines given to children and autism. I personally know parents that can pinpoint exactly which vaccine caused their kids to get autism. As a parent, having to look at yourself in the mirror and realize that you caused your child to get autism is a pretty sobering and devastating experience. The main narrative is that vaccines are safe and you don't want to let your children get sick. If you ever read those little inserts that are given for each vaccine, it lists all of the possible negative side effects that are known and they are not only a very long list, but also include all of the side effects that the "Anti Vax" group likes to talk about. This means that those companies know that an injury may occur. Anecdotally, if you look at the Amish people group, they are some of the healthiest individuals in America. With very little rates of autism and other major health and mental related issues, this can be attributed to not only not vaccinating, but also the way they live and the good foods they eat.

Each vaccine has some type of heavy metal in it like aluminum or mercury. This is to help the body have a bigger immune response to the injection. Some people claim heavy metal toxicity is a problem after the vaccines, as well as a destruction of the gut lining in the stomach. More true research needs to be released in this area, ideally by a third party that is not for or against vaccines.

If you decide to not vaccinate your children, it will be a little more difficult for you. If you live in big cities, all public schools, most private schools, and most day cares require them for your children to attend. To get around this, there are options such as a stay-at-home mom, homeschool, other private schools, and church schools. However, it seems that after the Covid shutdowns, parents have more and more people creating ways for schooling without vaccines. At this point in time, you should also be able to get medical or religious exemptions from vaccines by filling out forms and turning them into the schools. These are major family discussions and you should make your choices based on your own family needs.

For the sake of neutrality of this book, I will not suggest giving or not giving vaccinations to your kids, I am not a doctor. You should discuss with your spouse and pediatrician what is the best course of action. Keep in mind most people have biases for or against vaccines already. The goal is to make the best decision you can with as much information you can get. This includes doctors, friends, internet, ingredients lists, warning labels, etc. I was once told by someone that they trust the doctors "1000%." I just laughed to myself. I don't care what side of the aisle you sit on with any subject, but trusting someone that much which you don't know is not very smart. The whole idea of "science" is to actually question everything. Trusting is good, but blindly trusting is not good.

Chapter Twelve: When Does It Get Easier?

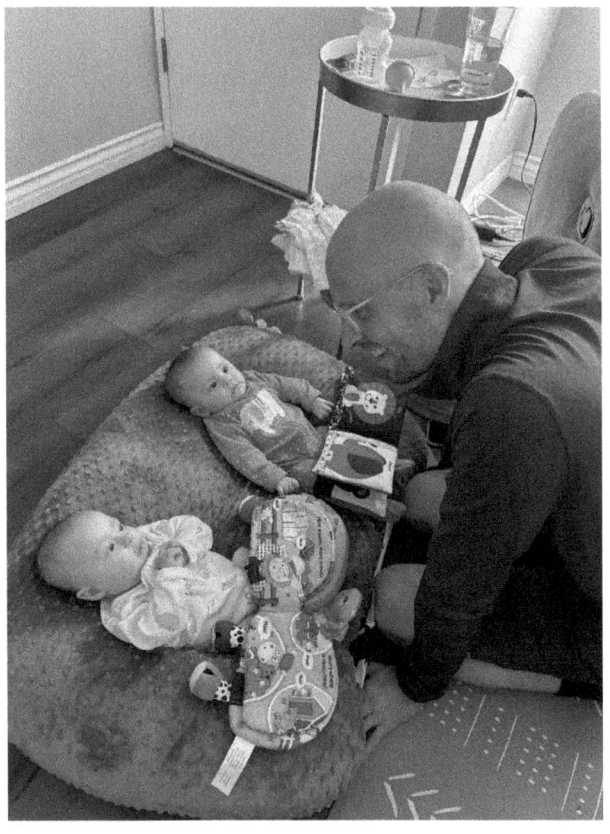

The short answer to when it gets easier is about 4-6 months, but just note that each season is a different type of hard. I will say though, it's not just super easy. At a certain point, the type of difficulty just changes into a new one. But when you finally get to sleep through the night again, aw man that is amazing!

Most parents notice a small reprieve at the 2-month mark, but at this 4–6-month time frame, the babies are sleeping more through the night and can go a little longer between feedings. They start giving little smiles and it's truly amazing. If you are blessed from the beginning with babies which sleep mostly through the night then thank Jesus for that blessing. As these babies grow and hit new little milestones, it gets easier.

Babies' eyesight will progress as they grow. Getting toys with dark contrasting colors (black, white and red) and having basic shapes and colors are great to start out with. Purchasing things to catch their attention like crib mobiles are also going to help them start to track back and forth. At the beginning they are not able to comprehend watching TV since their eyesight wasn't developed. I was able to get baby cuddle time while they napped and was able to catch up on some good shows.

The milestones are great to be a part of. It is not always fun for the babies though. Most babies hate tummy time and will protest or complain the whole time. Tummy time is important because it helps them strengthen their neck, arms, and backs so they are able to lift their heads up if they accidentally roll onto their tummy. Once they are strong enough and get it down, they will be rolling all over the place. It is a great feeling and makes you feel so proud when you see your baby's progress to the next phase.

Each new phase will be a "different hard." The hardest is at the beginning when they are very small and eat every few hours. Waking up and feeding them when you're already on a couple hours of sleep can be tough. Just keep going and at some point they will sleep longer. It's amazing when they go even one extra hour and you get just a little bit more sleep. But with each new milestone, your difficulty will change. What do I mean by that? It's difficult once they start rolling over, once they start eating solid foods, when they get sick for the first time, when they start to walk, and so on. The awesome thing is seeing them learn new skills and start to develop into the people they will one day become. Getting to be a part of that is such an amazing feeling that it is hard to describe.

Conclusion

Being a great husband and a twin Dad can be quite a daunting task. It is in all of us to be strong for our family. Sometimes we need help too, we are human after all. The great thing is that we typically love to provide for our family and always want to do what is best. Even with the ups and downs and frustrations, we push forward.

As men, we always need to be present for our families. Kids LOVE to play with Daddy. Their currency is not money, it's time and love. Spend time with them, tell them you love them. So many of us were never able to get that from our fathers. If that was you, now is the time to break the cycle and heal from your own past pains. Show your kids that you love them, even if it is difficult for you because this is what really matters. If you don't, then at the end of your life you will be saying how much more time you should have spent with the family. Most people regret not spending that time with them when they were more focused on trying to get that promotion or working the extra day to make an extra buck.

Your kids will grow up to be adults, but they aren't adults yet. Life will be hard and it's amazing when you have a father who is able to help you navigate through tough times. You can do this! Just remember to be patient and strong for your family. One day when your children are adults and understand life a little more, they'll say what an amazing dad you were. You'll be able to look back and reminisce with your wife and say "man, what a good life we've had."

Scott Southworth

Our Story

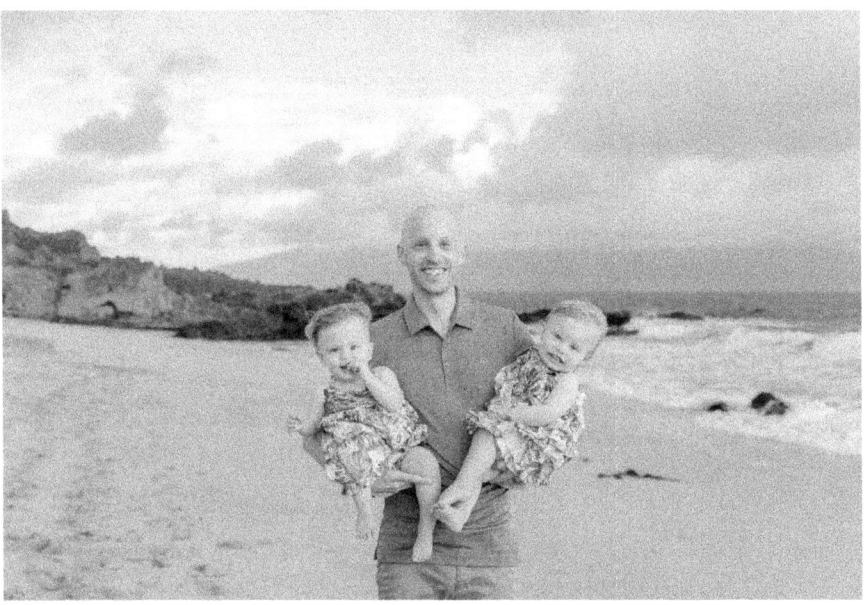

Hello, my name is Scott. For the purposes of this book, our journey started when we were having trouble conceiving. Now, some people try for years before they finally are able to get pregnant. However, after some research, we learned that after 1 year if you are doing everything correctly and still nothing has happened, then the chances of you conceiving without any help go down drastically. They say this because there could be some issue and if you don't fix that issue then you'll always struggle. So, my wife and I determined that after that 1-year mark we would go and seek some fertility help and found a very nice fertility doctor that was willing to help us out. She came highly recommended from someone that we know.

After many tests on both my wife and I, there were no definitive conclusions of why we were not able to conceive a baby. So, we were given two choices for help. The first was called Intrauterine Inception

(IUI), or to use a hormone called Clomiphene. IVF was not suggested to us just yet since we were still young and because the doctor believed that IVF should be the last resort. The IUI was going to cost us about $2,500 and the Clomiphene only $20 each round. However, with the Clomiphene, there is a higher chance of multiples as it makes MOM's body release multiple eggs at the same time. We chose Clomiphene mainly for financial reasons, but also because we didn't fully grasp the aspect of twins or triplets.

With the Clomiphene, we conceived twins on the first try. We almost conceived triplets! The doctors were able to see how many eggs my wife's ovaries released and confirmed three were released at that time. We were very happy to have our two awesome miracles. A lot of doctor's visits and a few months later we were told that one twin (twin B) was not growing as fast as the other one (Twin A). We were then referred to a high-risk doctor. With the current technology, they are able to get really close to approximate weights and lengths of all of the bones of the babies with good accuracy. This doctor was able to confirm that Twin B was indeed growing at a slower pace because there was a small umbilical cord flow problem. This high-risk doctor group had a few different doctors in their practice. At one appointment, one of the main doctors suggested to my wife that she could do something they called "Selective Reduction." This is just another term used for abortion of one twin to possibly help the other one. We were absolutely dismayed they would suggest killing one twin and asked to never see that specific doctor again. Looking back now, we can't imagine what life would be like without our second twin. She is so amazing and full of life.

Shortly after, tests revealed that Twin B was not growing well at all and that the babies may need to be born sooner rather than later. My wife was sent into the Antepartum section of the hospital at 25 weeks pregnant. What a crazy whirlwind of emotions that was. If you don't know much about pregnancy, a full term pregnancy is 40 weeks, and the doctors will only let twins go to about 36 weeks for safety reasons because they get too big after that. So, doing a little math, my wife was pretty early. At this point, both twins weren't weighing much more than 1 ½ pounds each. The hospital doctors gave my wife the Betamethasone steroid shot to help the babies' lungs mature a little bit faster just in case they had to be born soon. They ran tests a few times per day in order to check on the babies and make sure nothing bad was happening.

My wife stayed in the Antepartum department of the hospital for a total of seven weeks. This amount of time is highly unusual, but all of the tests for the babies were coming out positive so they decided that the babies were not needing to be born just yet. My wife really struggled there. I had to work during that time and would come and visit her on the weekends or if she needed me to give her a hug during the week because she was struggling mentally. She was the "talk of the town" though. She's very outgoing so she would walk around the floor with her big DJ headphones bobbing her head to worship music and loved making friends with all the nurses. She even met some of the other girls in the Antepartum section that were waiting to have their babies and became friends with them. Years later and they are still friends and talk all the time. .

At the Thirty-One weeks and five-day pregnancy mark one of the tests showed that the umbilical blood flow was reversing and that it was going to be more beneficial for Twin B to be born than it was to keep her inside. I was at home eating dinner at the time when I got a call from my wife and she put me on speaker phone when the nurse came in with the test results. I quickly packed a bag and headed for the hospital. We had about 10 hours after the results until the C-Section procedure.

When the twins were born they weighed 3 lbs 3 oz and 2 lbs 4 oz. We were told that they would spend two months in the NICU that would put them at that typical forty week full term mark. It was stressful yet peaceful for us. I guess because my wife had spent seven weeks at the hospital beforehand that helped. We also got the overwhelming peaceful feeling from God that no matter what happens while the babies were there, He would always be there for us and to trust Him. There were ups and downs while they were in the NICU, but we knew that no matter what happened, everything was going to be okay.

When babies were able to go home from an extensive stay in the NICU the nurses held a fun little graduation ceremony. It was hard for us to see the graduations of other babies while ours were still there, but we always were able to cheer for them. We still have been able to keep in contact with some of the families and nurses since we left. When our day came for graduation, we were happy and nervous at the same time. One of our twins was able to come home five days before the other twin. By day four, we had our routine down and were thinking it was going to be easy. Let me tell you that all of that changed when baby number two came home. When our second twin came home from the NICU it was so difficult. We barely got three hours of broken sleep each. We were pulling around the clock shifts and would wake the other napping parent up to help feed them. If you are able to get a routine down to where one parent can handle it while the other one sleeps, do it. We decided it was easier to have two hands on deck and decided the single option wasn't in our cards at the time, until we were able to start sleep training. Going through what we had to go through and all of the experiences that came along with it made me want to write a book to maybe, hopefully, help someone else in the future. I hope this book helps you in your journey and you love your twins and more kids as much as we love ours. Raising these kids is one of the best things that have ever happened in our lives and I couldn't imagine life not being a twin dad

The Ultimate Twin Dad Survival Guide

Random Advice and Food for Thought

Be the kind of dad you would want to have. Be patient, be friendly, be fun, be awesome. But remember, you are not their friend, you are their dad, their mentor, their role model. Make sure to be there for them

Time will go by more quickly than you think. Even when you're struggling, find a way to appreciate the now. Your little ones will not be this little for very long.

Try to put yourself in your kid's shoes. They do not know you had a bad day at work, they really just want to see you and spend time with you. Treat them well.

Be part of their daily routine and listen to them talk and talk about their day. Be excited for them.

Sometimes you have to go outside and tell God you are struggling and it's hard to keep going. Then, you go back inside and keep going.

Ephesians 6:4 in the bible – "Fathers, do not provoke your children to anger, but bring them up in the discipline and instruction of the Lord"

Your little one may appear to push your buttons on purpose and give off an attitude like an adult, but they still don't have the emotional maturity to be treated like one.

You're going to screw up and that's okay. Learn from it and fix it to prevent it from happening again.

Tell your children, "I like you," and "I'm proud of you." They need to hear these things too.

Don't expect anything to always go the way you want. You need to learn to roll with the punches and do the best you can.

Be the parent (or parents) that unconditionally believes in your children. They will be more successful in life if you are on their side.

Never have a favorite, love them both equally. Playing favorites will mess up a family forever.

A sense of humor is always required.

Let them play. Free play sparks kid's imaginations and development. Let them go outside, spin around in circles, play in the dirt, be loud when they can.

Your impatience becomes your child's anxiety. Your judgment becomes their self-doubt. Your disappointment becomes their shame. Your criticism becomes their inner voice. Your excitement becomes their excitement. Your love becomes their love. Your example becomes their life. Choose wisely.

Limit TV and screen time. So many studies have come out on how bad screen time for littles is a bad thing. Trust me, they'll learn to play with other toys if there are no screens.

Stand together with MOM. You and MOM are a team. Never let one parent say one thing and the other parent say something else. Never let secrets between the adults happen. Always stand beside each other's decision in front of the children and discuss amongst yourselves on the side and come to one single conclusion.

www.ingramcontent.com/pod-product-compliance
Lightning Source LLC
LaVergne TN
LVHW052048070526
838201LV00086B/5127